WIN

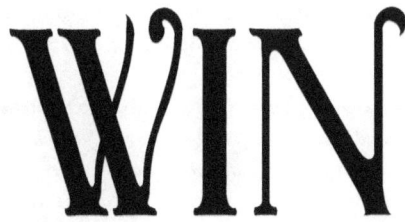

WIN

LIVING A VICTORIOUS
LIFE THROUGH JESUS CHRIST

REBECCA SORRELL

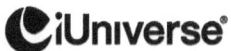

WIN
LIVING A VICTORIOUS LIFE THROUGH JESUS CHRIST

iUniverse books may be ordered through booksellers or by contacting:

iUniverse
1663 Liberty Drive
Bloomington, IN 47403
www.iuniverse.com
1-800-Authors (1-800-288-4677)

ISBN: 978-1-5320-6398-5 (sc)
ISBN: 978-1-5320-6403-6 (e)

Library of Congress Control Number: 2018914133

Print information available on the last page.

iUniverse rev. date: 11/29/2018

CONTENTS

To my children, Ronald and Amanda, who
have stood by my side in the home, hospital,
supermarket, gym, and park and through it all

Through the illness, the storm, the test, or whichever and
whatever you want to name it, they kept me energized and
hopeful and continuously told me, "You can walk again,
you can go back to work again, and you can live again."

Yes, I can. Yes, I can. And yes, I will.

Thanks!

Love, Mommy

INTRODUCTION

The Lord is in charge of my life. The true and living God put in my spirit to write a book and name it *Win*. It was February 21, 2017, at 3:47 a.m. The true and living God—the God of Abraham, Isaac, and Jacob—awakened me. I couldn't go back to sleep. So I obeyed God and started writing.

It's true what church family say, "God is going to get some glory out of this." So here is God's glory. I am giving him his glory by being obedient and writing this book. Praise him. Hallelujah! He is good all the time. His mercy and grace endure throughout all generations.

Jesus said in John 15:7 (NIV), "If you remain in me and my words remain in you ask whatever you wish, and it will be given you." So in other words, we win. Not maybe and not possibly. But we win! I stayed in God's Word day after day. I would pray, "Heavenly Father, please heal me. Please, King Jesus, allow me to walk again and give me back my health. I repent. I need you, God, every day." I had to repent, submit, and saturate myself in God and his Word.

I had to do like King David in the Bible. I asked God for mercy. In Psalms 51:1–2 (NIV), David begged for mercy when he committed adultery with Bathsheba. "Have mercy on me, O God, according to your great compassion blot out my transgressions. Wash away all my iniquity and cleanse me from my sin."

I had also sinned, but it wasn't like King David. I didn't take care of my health either. I was eating all the wrong foods late at night. I was not exercising, and on top of that, I would lay down after eating all that greasy food and go to sleep. I did that every night, a very bad habit. I had gained so much weight. I weighed 230 pounds. My blood pressure was also in the two hundreds. I was headed for Death Valley. I didn't take my health issues seriously.

Once I had my stroke, then I realized that I needed to change my eating and exercise habits. The day of my stroke, I started coughing up blood continuously, and the bathroom was spinning around and around.

I shouted out to my children, "Dial 9-1-1! I am having a stroke!"

My daughter got her cell phone and dialed 9-1-1. The paramedics rushed me to the hospital at Mansfield Methodist Hospital in Mansfield, Texas.

This book is a victory book. Reading God's Word daily motivated me and really encouraged me to take action and do it. James 2:17 (NIV) reads, "In the same way, faith by itself, if is not accompanied by action, is dead." Nike has a slogan that everyone is familiar with and knows very well. Just do it! That's exactly what I did. I activated Nike's slogan. I started writing, researching, and using my experience from my illness. I used all my tools.

I would like to present this to the church and the world, to inform everyone that, with God, you win. God is mighty. All power is in his hand. Heaven and earth belong to him. Everything in it is his. That means you and I belong to him.

Job 41:11 (NIV) reads, "Who has a claim against me that I must pay? Everything under heaven belongs to me." So with God on your side, you win. There is no losing, just winning. That's all God knows. All God does is win, win, win, and our hands go up and never come down.

Because we are winners, God doesn't lose. If you are a person who has had an illness, disease, hurt, or pain, you know firsthand what I am speaking about. Then repent, submit, and saturate yourself in God and his Word. I suggest you run to God swiftly. He is a strong tower. Watch him work on your behalf.

Psalm 18:1–2 (NIV) says, "I love you, O lord, my strength. The lord is my rock, my fortress and my deliverer; my god is my rock, in whom I take refuge. He is my shield and the horn of my salvation, my strong hold." And Psalm 61:3 (NIV) states, "For you have been my refuge, a strong tower; the righteous against the foe."

Proverbs 18:10 (NIV) reads, "The name of the lord is a strong tower; the righteous run to it and are safe." And Psalm 16:1 (NIV) says, "Keep me safe, O god, for in you I take refuge."

God cares for you. He is gracious and merciful. There is no one like him. You can search the world, but you will never find anyone else like him. He is Jehovah Rapha. This means "God heals you, the Lord our healer."

Psalm 147:3 (NIV) reads, "He heals the broken hearted and binds up their wounds." And Jeremiah 30:17 (NIV) states, "But I will restore you to health and heal your wounds, declares the lord, because you are called an outcast, Zion for whom no one cares."

Everyone needs to take some quality time out of his or her busy schedule every day and start reading God's Word instead of watching television for ten hours each day. When you are not watching television, you are on YouTube, Facebook, Instagram, Twitter, and Periscope for fourteen hours. I do not understand it. Please tell me. When do you sleep? Unless you are doing God's business and building up the kingdom and not tearing it down, then God will forgive you. Maybe God is trying to tell you to do something important, but you can't hear God because you are too busy. That's how a lot of people miss their blessings, by not recognizing God talking to them.

Start reading God's Word. You will feel so much better, and you will be blessed. Second Chronicles 7:14 (NIV) says,

> If my people, who are called by my name, will humble themselves and pray and seek my face and turn from their wicked ways, then will I hear from heaven and will forgive their sin and will forgive their sin and will heal their land.

Go ahead. Make an appointment with God. Pencil him in your day. Somewhere during your busy day, just stop everything. Block everyone out and give God ten, fifteen, twenty, thirty, or something. Give him some of your time because he gave you his only begotten Son who died on the cross for your sins.

That's the least you could do every day. Download the Bible app on your cell phone and then go to your calendar and make an appointment with God. Don't ever get too busy for God. He is the one who can heal you, so give him your mind, body, soul, and time. Search the Word and your heart. If you seek God, he will come through. You will win in the end. Trust me what I am telling you. I know what I am talking about. You will win.

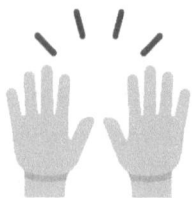

CHAPTER 1

THE STROKE

A stroke can make you or break your life. Your body can be 100 percent healthy one day, and the next day, you could be dialing 9-1-1 and have the paramedics transporting you to the hospital. Life can throw punches at you when you least expect it. Church family says that the devil brings sickness on you and Jesus heals you. Sometimes it's on us that brings sickness on ourselves.

John 10:10 (NIV) says, "The thief comes only to steal and kill and destroy; I have come that they may have life, and have it to the full." Psalm 118:17 (NIV) reads, "I will not die but live, and will proclaim what the lord has done."

When the physician says stroke, the patient normally replies, "A stroke? Would you please explain that to me?"

Statistics state that a stroke is the third-leading illness in America. The number-one illness is a heart attack, and number two is cancer. A stroke happens every forty seconds of the day. There are 795,000 new and recurrent ones each year. Approximately 160,000 people die from strokes every year, and 5 million survivors continue to suffer afterward. A stroke touches one out of ten families.

But with proper care, knowledge, and rehabilitation, stroke survivors can return home and continue their lives. There is life after a stroke. We know with God all things are possible. Matthew 19:26 (NIV) says, "Jesus looked at them and said, 'With man this is impossible, but with god all things are possible.'"

A stroke happens when the brain stops functioning. This permits an infarction or brain damage. The blood supply is stopped. The oxygen and nutrients never gets to the brain. This allows the artery to either be blocked or burst.

This damages a certain part of the brain, which no longer works as well as it did prior to the stroke. Normally the muscles and reflexes are all affected in the body. This, in turn, causes difficulty with walking, speaking, or feeling.

This is what happened to me. The stroke actively interfered with my mind, body, and soul. In other words, it impacted my life. The blood was trying to flow to my brain, and a blockage interrupted it.

A blood clot was blocking the blood flow. A blood clot is a buildup of fatty cholesterol deposits accumulating on the walls of your arteries. This translates into atherosclerosis (hardening of the arteries or high cholesterol). When a blood clot stops the blood from flowing in the blood vessels, the area is not getting the blood supply that it needs. The brain cells aren't watered, like a lawn that isn't nourished. So the brain cells die very quickly.

Eating Habits

If you are between five feet and five feet four inches, you should weigh 100 to 130 pounds. Of course, your age, condition, and nationality determines this. If you are anything over your proper height and weight, you need to start eating the correct foods and exercising. Lose the weight, so please stop all the fast food, drive-thru, and microwave dinners. Start eating healthy. Eat all the right foods, for instance, salad, vegetables, fruits, and whole grain wheats.

Have an apple instead of chips or a salad instead of a burger and fries, and drink eight glasses of water per day instead of soft drinks. Oh! Yes, please detox your mind every day and your body once a month. When detoxing your body, prepare eight ounces of water with lemon, lime, cucumber, and strawberries. Also you can drink eight ounces of water with a teaspoon of apple cider vinegar. Maybe go to the spa or sauna to remove toxins, whichever you choose to remove the toxins and reset your mind, body, and soul.

First Corinthians 6:19–20 (NIV) reads, "Do you not know that your body is a temple of the holy spirit, who is in you, whom you have received from god? You are not your own; you were bought at a price. Therefore, honor god with your body." Romans 12:1 (NIV) says, "Therefore, I urge you, brothers, in view of god's mercy, to offer your bodies as living sacrifices, holy and pleasing to god—this is your spiritual act of worship."

Therefore, if you develop healthy eating habits, you will have a healthy body, and you will live longer and look and feel better. Don't forget to exercise. That's just as important as eating healthy. Go for a walk each day for about thirty minutes. They go hand in hand, just like peanut butter and jelly. Eating healthy and exercising equals a healthy long life. Thank you, Jesus!

You can stop a stroke before it happens by losing weight. You can reduce it by 40 percent. That's almost half of what's expected of a high-risk person. African Americans and Hispanics are at a high risk for a stroke. The following are a combination for a stroke: hypertension, high cholesterol, obesity, and diabetes. These factors are common among these two nationalities. Stop consuming so much alcohol, sugar, salt, and carbs. For morning and afternoon snacks, consider two pieces of fruit, veggies, and a small handful of nuts. Keep track of your food, and eat the correct amount.

Menu

Saturday	Breakfast	Lunch	Dinner
	Strawberry smoothie	Bowl of veggie soup and half sandwich	3–4 ounces salmon, veggies, and small salad
Sunday	Fruit smoothie with half-cup plain lowfat yogurt	Bowl of veggie soup and half sandwich	3–4 ounces grilled chicken, veggies, and small salad
Monday	Berry smoothie with half-cup plain lowfat yogurt	3 ounces chicken and half-cup chopped veggies	3–4 ounces fish, veggies, and half-cup brown rice
Tuesday	Oatmeal and a banana	3 ounces tuna and half-cup chopped veggies	3–4 ounces grilled chicken, veggies, and half-cup brown rice
Wednesday	Oatmeal and a peach	3–4 ounces turkey meat and half-cup veggies	3–4 ounces stir-fried shrimp and veggies
Thursday	Whole wheat toast, two eggs, and an apple	3 ounces smoked salmon and half-cup veggies	3–4 ounces lean steak and small salad
Friday	Breakfast burrito (whole wheat wrap, half-cup black beans, and eggs) and a bowl of grapes	3 ounces turkey meat, half-cup veggies, and two slices whole wheat bread	"Treat Dinner!" Fill your plate with whatever you want

CHAPTER 2

BLOOD OF JESUS (BLOOD FLOW)

Praises include "covered by the blood," "There's power in the blood," "the blood of Jesus," "The blood of Jesus will never lose its power," "The blood of Jesus protects us," and "the precious blood of the Lamb of God." These are essential when you finally regain consciousness after you have lost the flow of blood going through your body. This is when Jesus steps into your situation and begins to turn things around. At this point, you then begin to feel forgiven and cleansed. Once the blood starts flowing again through your body, a feeling of restoration is circulating through your veins.

Oxygen is very important to the brain. Without oxygen, the brain cannot function. Its electrochemical process will not work. If there is no oxygen, you will lose consciousness within five to ten seconds. This, in turn, creates brain damage within minutes. This is what happened to me on the morning of my stroke. The room started spinning around and around.

Whether you donate blood or instantly notice yourself bleeding, whatever the person's reaction, it is literally a carrier of life. Think of it as a transporter that carries food to our cells. If you put a drop of blood under a microscope, you would see plasma, the liquid that holds the blood cells and gives blood its consistency. Red blood cells (corpuscles) hold the food. The cells also contain oxygen and other nutrients like glucose, a chemical that the body needs to survive.

The red blood cells feed the different organs and then go through the veins to carry the leftovers to the heart. The blood cells are where the red color come from. On the other hand, the white blood cells are called "infection fighters." Guess what they do. That's correct. They fight infection. When infection or inflammation threatens the body, white blood cells increase in number to fight the infection. Next, the platelets are responsible for clotting. For instance, if you were to have a cut somewhere on your body, the platelets form a web that traps other blood cells to stop the flow of blood.

Annual Checkup

I didn't schedule a time or have time to go to my primary doctor to renew my medicine. I also wasn't taking my medicine according to the directions on the bottles. I relied on my own judgment when it was time to take it. I made bad decisions about my health. So I basically helped create my own stroke by not taking care of myself. I told myself, *I don't need this medicine. I am young. I am not old. Medication is for older individuals, not young ones.*

Of course, I stopped taking it, and you saw what happened. I had a stroke. Don't copy my example. If you do, then you will have what I had, a stroke. Remember, keep your doctor appointments. Try not to cancel or put them on hold until later. Your appointments are necessary when it's concerning your health.

If you must use vacation, paid time off, sick leave, or personal time, then use one of your days. Just go. Don't ignore or reschedule the appointment. You should prioritize this as mandatory in your calendar or on your cell phone. Once a year, you are supposed to see your primary physician to receive your annual checkup updates. Maybe this year he or she will check all your important functions in your body. By doing this, you will know what is and is not working properly.

This why you have medical insurance deducted from your paycheck once a month. During your checkup, your doctor will check your blood pressure and weight and test your blood. There's a possibly that all three of these could be in the danger zone. You need to continue to do this as you increase with age. I didn't keep my yearly doctor appointment. Therefore, I am suggesting that you take care of your health.

However, your doctor can recognize when a red light is flashing and a stroke is about to occur in your life.

Your doctor will tell you, "Hello! Listen to me! Your blood pressure, weight, and blood tests are in the danger zone. Change your eating habits and exercise. You do know that you are what you eat."

Therefore, your doctor can stop a stroke before it begins. Thank God for the medical occupations because, with God and medical employees, we have life. That's what my primary physician was trying to tell me, but I ignored his advice.

I would say, "I'm healthy. I don't need to do all that. I am still young."

Remember, don't do as I do, but do as I say. Keep your annual checkups and listen to your doctor's advice. Once again, take care of your health.

CHAPTER 3

MY MIND (MY BRAIN)

Isaiah 26:3 (NIV) reads, "You will keep in perfect peace him whose mind is steadfast, because he trusts in you." The brain is fascinating. It needs oxygen to survive like a car needs gasoline. Messages travel by electrical impulses and by releasing chemicals (neurotransmitters).

But when there is an interruption, for instance, a stroke, some of the brain cells are damaged. Therefore, messages don't get through because of damages to the brain, such as neurons being damaged, which creates imbalances and changes in mood and thoughts.

Strokes start in a different area of the body, and while traveling to the brain, this is the part that gets affected. The brain is made up of various parts. The cerebellum next to the spinal cord was the area where I had my stroke. The brain has 100 billion nerve cells. Colossians 3:2 (NIV) reads, "Set your minds on things above, not on earthly things."

The pons area of the brain is responsible for muscle tone, reflex actions, and alertness. The cortex is responsible for mobility and sensations. This is where we learn to walk, understand, and communicate. This is what makes us humans. We can form relationships and solve complex problems. Having a stroke in this area will affect your speech, memory, personality, sensations, and strengths.

The mental process in my brain was affected. When the blood clot stopped the blood flow and my cerebellum was damaged, this also impacted the pons and the cortex of my brain. So I had a left-brain stroke.

Left-Brain Stroke

So I had a left-brain stroke, which means that the left side of my brain was affected. The cells in the cerebellum was damaged. The left side of my brain, the pons and cortex, was affected. Also the frontal lobe of my brain was damaged. This area controls your movement and decision making, such as planning, organizing, and memorizing.

The left hemisphere of the brain is responsible for language, reading, writing, calculations, and communication. Where a stroke happens, for example, the left or right hemisphere, is very important. Whichever side you had the stroke on will determine that the opposite side would be weak. Therefore, you will have to strengthen the weak side.

Also a left hemisphere stroke can cause depression. That's why I kept myself busy in God's Word or had plans with a full agenda each day. Daily, I would take time to talk to God through prayer. I would detox and reset my mind, keeping it clean from strong hold. I would limit items like television, telephone, and certain conversations.

I would keep my mind on Jesus, remain focused, and try not to get off course. I would also go work out at the gym by lifting weights, trying to strengthen my right side, which was weak. On January 5, 2017, I started at Tarrant County College in continuing education, receiving certificates in office assistant I and office assistant II. So my mind has been occupied. I try to stay strong by strengthening my skills and my right side. When my right side gets weak, I must use my cane to help my right side.

CHAPTER 4

DIFFERENT STROKES FOR DIFFERENT FOLKS

A small percentage of patients have a transient ischemic attack (TIA), actually only 15 percent. TIAs are normally ignored. This is what I had at first, but try to guess what happened. That's correct. I ignored it because it was instantly. The patient will recognize that he or she just had a TIA, but this is where the problem is created.

Then they ignore it because it happens so rapidly, within fifteen minutes, until the patient just continues with what he or she is doing like nothing has happened. And then boom! It becomes worse. There's blurred vision, numbers, weakness, or paralysis of the hand, arm, or face. This is a red flag warning. Your body is telling you to take care of yourself. You need to call 9-1-1 or immediately go to the emergency room. Try your best to prevent a stroke.

Next is the thrombotic or thrombosis. This is where the blood clot stops the blood flow in the brain or neck. This is what I had happen to my brain. The blood was trying to travel to my brain but couldn't because of a blood clot, another name for atherosclerosis, a buildup of cholesterol deposits in the blood.

Thick deposits of fat forms, and the passageway is too narrow for the blood to flow through. Instead the blood forms a clot, or embolism.

Eventually the blood clot breaks off a piece and travels to the brain or neck, where the arteries are smaller. The blood clot gets stuck and stops blood from flowing past the embolism.

Last is the hemorrhagic stroke. This stroke can be deadly. Because of hypertension, this is how it starts, which results in ruptures, spilling blood into the brain. High blood pressure can be the root cause of this. Just like a car gets overheated, a person's blood pressure can reach its peak. So stay cool and calm always, and live a healthy lifestyle.

That's all I have to say about types of strokes. Just remain healthy, and use your five senses God gave you. Common sense is all you need. You know your body, so when it tries to tell you something, "Listen!"

CHAPTER 5

THE HOSPITAL

I was transported to Mansfield Methodist Hospital, one of the top hospitals in the Dallas/Fort Worth area. At the hospital, I was informed that I had a left-brain stroke. A tremendous amount of information that caused the stroke was revealed. Strokes don't come out of nowhere. There are warning signs. You just must recognize them and receive treatment before it's too late!

I had an embolic action where the blood clots with a mass of tissue, blood, and cholesterol. The clot begins somewhere else in the body and starts clotting probably in the neck area, possibly the cerebellum. Therefore, blood can't flow. It is stopped in the neck area, and the cells are damaged. It affects either the left or right side of the brain. Because the blood is not feeding the cells, oxygen is stopped and can't get to the brain.

Blood clots are usually the result of other problems that affect the normal flow of blood, such as atherosclerosis, which is the hardening of the arteries, caused by high cholesterol. I was in the hospital for two weeks. The staff was extremely nice. My physician is an awesome doctor. My pressure was in the two hundreds.

After they reduced my pressure to normal, 120/80, then my doctor requested brain and heart scans. I had a left-brain stroke. My right side was affected. This is my dominant side. I am right-handed. The hospital did an echocardiogram (EKG), which is useful for detecting the heart as a source of an embolus. An EKG is a device that is placed on the patient's chest or neck, and sound waves bounce off the heart or neck. The sound waves are recorded. If there is a blood clot, then the machine can draw a picture of the problem.

Another test my doctor requested was a computerized tomography (CT) in order to obtain specific information about my stroke. A patient lies down inside a giant white doughnut, and the CT takes pictures of the inside of the brain.

Last my physician requested a magnetic resonance imaging (MRI), which provides a more detailed picture type and location of the stroke. It is a super-conducting magnet creating a powerful force with radio frequency taking pictures of the brain. A MRI is particularly good at looking at the brain stem and cerebellum.

While I was waiting for the results, I was looking at Bible scriptures on my cell phone. Psalms 41:3 (NIV) reads, "The lord will sustain him on his sickbed and restore him from his bed of illness." And Jeremiah 17:14 (NIV) says, "Heal me, o lord, and I will be healed; save me and I will be saved, for you are the one I praise." Family and friends came to visit me which was nice to see everyone.

Walk It Out

So when I tried to walk, especially my right leg, which was extremely weak, it was very upsetting for me. I would walk up and down the hallway of the hospital to strengthen my legs. I continued to walk with a limp. The nurse had to go get me a walker. I would walk every day with the walker to the end of the hall and back to my hospital room.

Two areas of the brain can affect our balance and movement. The blood clot affected my cerebellum, which coordinates my every movement. It helps me keep my balance. So because my cerebellum was affected, my balance was off. The cerebellum coordinates the speech muscle movements, but my speech was not affected, thank God. Second Corinthians 5:7 (NIV) says, "We live by faith, not by sight." And 2 Corinthians 5:7 (KJV) reads, "for we walk by faith, not by sight."

Hebrews 11:6 (NIV) states, "And without faith it is impossible to please god, because anyone who comes to him must believe that he exists and that rewards those who earnestly seek him." Hebrews 11:1 (NIV) says, "now faith is being sure of what we hope for and certain of what we do not see." And Romans 10:17 (NIV) states, "consequently, faith comes from hearing the message, and the message is heard through the word of Christ."

I had to use these faith scriptures in the Bible to help me strive to walk again. I had to say Bible verses repeatedly, hoping that each time I would get better at walking. The two weeks I was in the hospital, the staff was terrific and amazing. They worked well with my disability.

The rehabilitation staff suggested that I receive more therapy, so I replied yes. The staff informed my insurance benefit coordinator that I needed more therapy, and I was approved. My records were sent to Centre for Neuro Skills, located in Irving, Texas, an excellent rehabilitation program.

CHAPTER 6

STROKE SYMPTOMS

There are symptoms of a stroke. For instance, balance relates to difficulty walking and coordination (better known as vertebrobasilar insufficiency). Look for poor blood flow to the brain stem. There is an intermittent vertebral artery, or a damaged cerebellum. You will feel a sense of weakness in muscles with your leg, arm, or face. When the body isn't active, muscles weaken. Another one is paralysis, which takes place during a stroke.

The face droops and appears nonsymmetrical when talking and smiling. This is caused by a lack of oxygen to the face. Also your speech becomes slurred and noticeable. You have trouble speaking and understanding the spoken word. Your intelligent words become difficult. Next, a stroke may affect your vision. You will have trouble seeing or not seeing clearly. A patient can experience double vision or blind spots. A stroke survivor may have cells destroyed in the visual cortex.

A stroke can create poor understanding. A stroke survivor will have difficulty understanding certain subjects such as statements or commands. The stroke patient who is engaged in a conversation will have trouble receiving communication. Throughout the conversation, the patient will look confused or lethargic as if it didn't register with the brain.

Everyone knows that headaches are common with strokes. Migraines or severe headaches come after a stroke. A person will admit that the migraines is so painful after a stroke. It feels like a sharp pain piercing your head, like someone hitting you with a hammer on your head.

Losing sensation is another symptom that happens after a stroke. Maybe your legs or arms have no feelings. They're just numb. It could be damaged nerves, causing your senses to probably be affected. For instance, your smell, taste, and hearing don't function normally like they used to. Becoming dizzy, or vertigo, is normal before a stroke. The patient will have problems with balancing. The back of the brain is affected, where the vertebral and basal arteries reside.

So the patient will have complications with sitting or walking. The stroke patient feels like the entire house is spinning around. His or her equilibrium is off, and he or she becomes nauseous and starts vomiting. Last, reflexes are affected after a stroke. When a stroke patient eats his or her food, this person will have trouble swallowing and sometimes gag. The patient reflex is not as efficient as before the stroke.

Blood Pressure

You need to have your blood pressure taken frequently to prevent strokes or heart attacks. Also you need to exercise to start your blood circulating to help elevate your pressure. Your blood pressure is what keeps your blood flowing and moving in a rhythmic way through your arteries. When taking your blood pressure, there are two numbers on the blood pressure machine. The top is the systolic reading. This is when your heart squeezes and contracts to push the blood through your arteries. This keeps your blood moving.

The bottom number is the diastolic reading. This is when the heart rests between beats. Regular blood pressure is written as 120/80 or 120 over 80. Write it however you wish, but make sure you write it correctly. This is normal pressure, so remember the two numbers. If the top number is high or over 120, then this means that the heart must work harder to push the blood through your arteries.

If the bottom number is high or over 80, then this means that the heart remains elevated between beats. Don't allow your blood pressure reading to rise too high or go below regular readings because high blood pressure is just as bad as low blood pressure. And vice versa. Keep watch on your pressure.

Bad and Good Cholesterol

Your body manufactures cholesterol (triglycerides) (fats) for functions, but there is bad cholesterol and good cholesterol. There are two blood cholesterol levels: high-density lipoprotein (HDL) and low-density lipoprotein (LDL). Lipoprotein carries cholesterol in the blood. When you go to your physician for your annual checkup, ask him or her to check your cholesterol level readings in order to inform you about how much bad cholesterol is in your blood.

HDL prevents you from a stroke or heart attack. High LDL can lead to serious health problems such as clogged arteries or heart disease. You need to lower your LDL and change your lifestyle in order to improve your LDL. Cholesterol is found in meats, cheese, milk, and margarine. These four items contribute to higher cholesterol levels. Too much of these contributions leads to trouble. Lipoprotein is a substance of fat protein produced by the liver.

The lipoprotein that does most of the work is the LDL cholesterol. After the LDL has given your body what it needs, the LDL is still

17

floating around in your body with nowhere to go. Eventually this LDL settles on your artery walls, clogging passageways or creating clots that break off and travel to the brain. That is why the LDL is referred to as bad cholesterol.

HDL, on the other hand, carries cholesterol back to the liver for elimination. HDL sucks up the leftover cholesterol to try to help clear up the arteries. High cholesterol comes from enormous amounts of LDL in the blood. Lower your cholesterol intake in order to prevent strokes. If you lower your LDL, 40 percent of strokes will decrease by 25 percent. If your LDL is more than 100 mg/dl, then you should be on medication. Your LDL should read under 200 mg/dl. Please get your LDL to 70 mg/dl, a normal reading, by eating healthy and exercising.

CHAPTER 7

LEFT-BRAIN STROKE

I am going to discuss left-brain stroke because that's what I am familiar with. So all the symptoms I had with the left-brain stroke is like the right-brain stroke. With a left-brain stroke, everything on the right side is affected and vice versa. If you had a right-brain stroke, then everything on the left side is affected. Although you have some weakness on your right side from your left-brain stroke, you can gradually strengthen your weakness by going to the gym to lift weights, do cardio, and exercise the weak side.

The left hemisphere of the brain controls most of our basic language skills. Your vocabulary will become affected. Maybe you may not be able pick up the conversation. There is a possibility that you will use a type of gesture with your hands while trying to speak. Also your visual memory will become confused. For example, when you read your daily emails, there is a chance that you don't remember what you read within the next five minutes.

Nevertheless, impaired judgement, for instance, sensory impairment, memory loss, attention deficient, time deficiency, and abstract reasoning, are all disorders of impairment. Basically, a left-brain stroke patient's judgement is poor. It's off on the wrong track. A stroke survivor may drive without his or her driver's license or eyeglasses, or the sense of directions are not clear. It is dangerous to the stroke patient and everyone else.

Emotions play a big part in a stroke patient's life. You may go from crying to laughing. In the right-brain stroke patient, it is more extreme than the left-brain stroke patient. Medicine can help with this. It can shift your mood imbalance quickly. With time, understanding and researching your illness can help.

Neuron Recover

Your neurons will return and become active again. Neurons find an alternative way or another route to implement. Once they are damaged, they become new and go a different direction. You can also recover by retraining yourself through a program. Also use God's Word in your life, and maybe your life will become different than before. You can have a full life; it's just different than before.

You will also have communication disabilities. The left side of your brain controls your communication, like language, comprehension, logic, and rational thinking. It works in coherence with the right side of your brain. Therefore, these skills are affected from either a left- or right-brain stroke. After a stroke, your speech may come out different. You will have language disabilities. Your words may be slurred so your words will not be understood, or your pronunciation may not be clear.

In a left-brain stroke patient, depression is more common. Your words will not come out as they should. For example, one word becomes difficult in the sentence that you are trying to communicate. That one word will have rearranged the entire conversation. Language disabilities will broaden in left-brain stroke patients. You might have to point to something instead of speaking.

A rehabilitation program can help you reconstruct your communication. At first, maybe you can just communicate with two- or three-word phrases. With time and practice on sentence structures again and again, eventually you will begin to complete sentences by reading and writing clearly.

Paralysis on the Right Side of the Body

Whether you have had a left- or right-brain stroke, your weakness will be on the opposite side of your body. I had a left-brain stroke, so my paralysis, or weakness, was on my right side, but I remain in God's Word.

With time and a rehabilitation program, a stroke patient can improve rapidly when a stroke survivor regains consciousness from the dizziness from the stroke. This is the part where the blood cannot flow to your brain and you are not getting any oxygen.

But when you regain consciousness, that's when you realize that you cannot move your right or left side or your leg or arm is very weak. It just depends which side of the brain you had your stroke.

The weakness is like dead weight. You can recover by remaining in God's Word with proper rehabilitation and medication. Daily living will become a chore, like getting dressed. When you have a disruption in the brain, it causes problems with everyday living. You can't move like you once did before the stroke. The daily activities will shorten because you can't perform like before.

Depression

A left-brain stroke can cause depression. An estimated 15 to 40 percent experience depression, and 70 percent of left-brain stroke patients have depression. Successful rehabilitation and antidepressant medication can help improve depression symptoms. Depression can be a result of a loss of brain chemicals that the brain injury damages.

Here is a list: continuous sadness, change in appetite, fewer activities, irritability, distant communication, less concentration, sleep disorder, and loss of self-esteem. Depression is a serious medical illness. It's how you think and act, along with your behavior, like feeling sad or having a depressed mood. The patient may feel hopeless or unimportant or is sometimes unable to live a normal life, especially when you lose your job or can no longer work a job. This involves the mind, emotions, thoughts, feelings, behavior, and sense of well-being.

When a person has extended periods of unhappiness or hopeless as well as senses of having no future, the patient loses interest in activities that he or she once enjoyed. The patient has a mood disorder, which includes guilt, anger, or feelings of shame. Also the patient experiences relationship difficulties, reduced energy, or poor concentration. The patient may complain more or say he or she is always in pain. Depression is treatable. Psychotherapy and support groups will help patients accept major changes in their life.

CHAPTER 8

WHAT HAPPENS

What makes a rehabilitation successful is providing information about what happened on the day of the stroke and why. Proper diagnosis is needed to help prevent a stroke from happening again. The rehabilitation centers need to know exactly what happened. Did the patient faint, or what was the patient doing? Did the patient have a headache, or did he or she feel numbness? These questions and others will help determine what type of treatment is needed.

My information concerning my stroke was that I was age fifty-two. I am an African-American female. I had a prior TIA. I had hypertension and high cholesterol. I was overweight. I was working overtime at a job. I was not taking medicine as directed. I was getting dressed for work and experienced immediate dizziness. I started coughing up blood and called 9-1-1.

The rehabilitation staff will concentrate on the patient's abilities, not just inabilities. They will determine their strengths and weaknesses and which equipment that will be helpful to the patient. What can the person do now? What are the patient's long- and short-term goals? Is there is anything that would hinder the individual's progress? The staff will make the decision on the type of treatment that is right for the patient.

Rehabilitation is vital to your health and improvement. This is done by implementing and reinforcing structure. A combination of high blood pressure, high cholesterol, and blood thinner medications along with occupational, physical, and speech therapy will help you regain your strength. I will go further into details in chapter 9 about each one of these areas to a renewed life.

I went to Health South, located in Arlington, Texas, the first rehabilitation center after two weeks in the hospital. I was at Health South for two weeks. The staff asked if I wanted more therapy. I replied yes. My records were then transferred to Centre for Neuro Skills, located in Irving, Texas. This was my second rehabilitation. I was there for two weeks. I was an outpatient; I wasn't a resident at the center.

I was dropped off at 9:00 a.m. and picked up at 2:00 p.m. Both rehabilitation centers have helped me totally. They are similar in technique but different in skills. I thank God for the two rehabilitation centers. Praise God. Stroke patients can forget information. That's normal after having a stroke. You could tell them about your day at school or work. The next second, they will not remember what you talked about. Most patients have a problem processing information. This is associated with left frontal lobe damage.

Why It Happened

It was a physical condition with me. In previous chapters, I mentioned that I was engaging in all the wrong behaviors that helped to create the disease. I was consuming all the wrong foods, eating late-night meals and sleeping afterwards, not taking my medication as directed, and not exercising. These were the factors why it happened.

The result of this is a clogged artery leading to my brain. That's why my doctor requested various tests at the hospital to have information about my left-brain stroke. I had received cell damage in the back of my brain (where the cerebellum is located). Another area was on my left side of my brain (left lobal area). Third and last was at the top left of my brain (parietal lobe). Understanding the factors of what happened and why has enlightened my mental ability. These factors will also help the staff at the rehabilitation centers.

CHAPTER 9

REHABILITATION

At Health South, the staff implemented activities. Strength and recovery were their main goals, specifically trying to strengthen my weak side to recovery. Then transferred me to my family at home. Centre for Neuro Skills was concerned with putting me back into society with different capabilities to a renewed life. There are different staff members at rehabilitation. Every morning I had physical therapy at 9:00 a.m. A rehabilitation nurse and rehabilitation doctor was assigned to each patient.

The nurse administered the medicine every day before breakfast. The dietician would create the menu for breakfast, lunch, and dinner. A stroke patient's nutritional needs change, and a need for a special diet for elimination of waste from the digestive tract was necessary. The doctor would check daily to maintain accurate records so that everything was going well toward recovery.

The doctor was the leader of the group. I had a neurologist, who I would see on regular visits when I first recovered. His office was at Mansfield Methodist Hospital. He was concerned about my brain and behavior. He would perform tests or ask me questions pertaining to my stroke. This was to evaluate cognitive abilities, behavioral problems, and psychological structure. Every day after taking my medicine and eating breakfast in my room, I would clean up and dress for physical therapy.

Health South would promote independence. A stroke patient has to complete a task with minimal help. This included my ability to bathe, brush my teeth, comb my hair, dress myself, sit in a chair, walk with a cane, groom myself, walk, go grocery shopping, and perform duties at home. Each one of these chores became difficult. We often take these things for granted. To have a stroke patient take the necessary steps to perform these chores are time consuming. The staff would determine my daily progress.

From putting on my pants to tying my shoe was demanding. It's better if you have elastic at the top of your pants. Zippers are irritating to a stroke patient. Pullover shirts are easier than button-up shirts. Clothes should be loose fitting. It's better if you sit in a chair when putting on your clothes. Electric shavers are better than razor blades. Taking a shower must be broken down into a chain of events, from turning on the water to wetting and applying soap to the washcloth.

The goal of going through rehabilitation is independence. Have the stroke patient do these tasks himself or herself with minimal assistance. It doesn't matter how long it takes the patient, as long as he or she regains independence.

Physical Therapy

The physical therapy staff at Health South would come to each patient's room and have everyone walk, either with a walker or cane, or get pushed in a wheelchair to the exercise room for our daily workout. The physical therapist is concerned with your motor function. The therapist concentrates on your walking ability, balance, and coordination. The therapist focuses on strength, endurance, and posture. The strategy is to build hope for the future.

The first year, many patients continue to make progress. Researchers state that 70 percent of stroke survivors become independent in their daily living. This independence transforms into confidence, which helps with motivating and keeping hope alive. We all know that with God all things are possible, such as independence, confidence, and motivation. Physical therapy is different for various parts of the body.

My right side was weakened from the stroke. So the physical therapist focused on strengthening my right side. If you don't enhance the weak muscles, then spasticity sets in. This means the imbalance of muscles, tension, and movement. The stroke survivor could have swelling and pain in his or her legs. Various methods of therapy are needed.

When a person has a stroke, the strong muscles become weak. They need to be strengthen and toned. A stroke creates inactivity, which in turn makes the person take frequent breaks throughout the day.

Weights and Strength

Physical therapy exercises enhance overall performances. A patient needs to learn to move about freely to obtain full independence, whether it is with a wheelchair, walker, or cane. A stroke patient with severe motor dysfunction has communication problems, for example, decision making. Fortunately with all the damage the stroke has created, muscles, balance, and spasticity can be reversed.

Exercise with weights to build your muscles. Make sure you put the weights on your weak leg to make it stronger. Use balance techniques to reverse poor muscle tone and weakness. This could result from leaning too much on one side.

The physical therapist would put us in groups to count as we lifted the weights. I would do stretch exercises on the mat in the exercise room. They would try to make me use the treadmill, but I wasn't ready. The therapist would suggest that I walk up and down the halls with my walker. Sometimes I would walk along the parallel bars.

Spastic Leg

When there is a malfunction in the passageway in the brain triggered by a stroke, the malfunction resists passive motion. This is spasticity. When you try to put on your pants and your leg won't move in the desired direction, the result is a tightness in your leg. Spasticity can make your leg appear frozen. You must exercise to improve spasticity. Spasticity and paralysis exist together.

When a stroke person has spasticity, this individual tries to bend his or her leg. Normally if it is tight or stiff like a board, you must loosen the tightness. By doing the range of motion exercises by relaxing your muscles, to have a proper body position and improved muscle function, learn to move on a spastic leg.

Braces

Different treatment and support equipment are needed for weak muscles and a spastic leg. Braces, ankle support, and shoe inserts keep joints stable. Sometimes a stroke survivor has trouble with walking. Because this person can't lift his or her foot, the name for this is drop foot. The muscles are weak in the ankle. The patient may need an ankle brace to support it and help him or her walk better and have correct posture. Also the stroke patient needs special shoes, preferably tennis shoes. These are better because they are nonslip.

Shoes

I went out and purchased a four of pairs of Skechers tennis shoes. I like them because they help me balance as I walk. They provide support, which I need. If a stroke patient has spasticity and wants to purchase other shoes other than tennis shoes, then go online. When purchasing tennis shoes or another type of shoes, make sure they have a lot of support and are comfortable. Ensure they are easy to slip on and take off. You need proper shoes to walk correctly and have stability in your posture. This is very important so you won't lose your balance and fall. The recovery from a fall would be intense. Thank God, I haven't fallen. The Lord keeps me balanced.

Using a cane and shoes with support will have a stroke patient on the road to recovery. A stroke patient may start walking with a quad base cane that has four legs. As progress continues, then he or she will transfer to a standard cane. This makes the stroke survivor feel confident.

Floors

Walking on carpet apparently is much more dangerous then wood. The thickness of the carpet slows your mobility, whereas wood floors enhance your mobility. Also climbing stairs can become difficult. When climbing stairs or walking up the curb, use the unaffected leg first. Remember, "up with the good leg and down with the bad leg."

Making Progress

Both rehabilitations at Health South and Centre for Neuro Skills have helped me tremendously. Both concentrated on developing a stroke patient's walking ability. The therapist had myself and the other patients use weights and do exercises. We walked up and down sidewalk curbs and stairs. We used parallel bars, treadmill, and bicycles. At Centre for Neuro Skills, the therapist eventually removed the walker from me. The therapist introduced me to the four-quad cane and then transferred me to the standard cane.

The staff would encourage the stroke patients to the next level. At Centre for Neuro Skills, the therapist would massage my leg to prevent spasticity. The therapist would relax my muscles to loosen them and to build better mobility in my legs. The therapist motivated me entirely to the point that I was becoming satisfied with both rehabilitations. They retained accurate records of my daily progress. This, in turn, had me repeating phrases like "God is good all the time, and all the time God is good!" and "I can do all things through Christ who strengthens me." Thank you, Jesus.

Occupational Therapy

Occupational therapy is a rehabilitation program of daily living. It's to retrain stroke patients in memory capabilities in their movement and coordination and to improve their activities of daily living, such as eating, getting dressed, cooking, cleaning house, taking showers, brushing teeth, driving a car, and doing the shopping at the supermarket. These activities we do daily. Because a stroke patient has some impairment, the daily living chores are limited, and they become a chore.

The therapist implements ideas on retraining and reteaching everyone. These activities must be mastered. The therapist will supervise the patient to a restored normal life, whereas before a stroke patient could multitask each one of these activities. After a stroke, one activity is equivalent to two activities. They become twice as hard, but it takes patience and strength as long as the stroke survivor does it himself or herself. Rehabilitation centers refer to this as independence, and that's what occupational therapist are trying to promote, independence.

Real-Life Training

Health South has a layout of a real world design at the center. There are rooms divided into real life in order for you to practice for that day when you have successfully completed the process and finished your recovery at rehabilitation. Once you have entered the real world and transition back into real life, it's a carbon copy of real life. One room has a supermarket (with food on the shelves), a cash register, and a car in a parking space with additional parking spaces beside it. Another room has a kitchen with cabinets, refrigerator, sink, stove, and food.

This enables the patient to focus on self-awareness. It welcomes him or her to the real world but under close supervision by staff members. As the patient participates in each scenario, the therapist grades accordingly, and the patient becomes more confident. The patient will be able to handle more responsibility when he or she goes home. This will motivate the patient to finish and succeed with the rehabilitation program.

At Centre for Neuro Skills Rehabilitation, occupational therapy was different in their program. It wasn't a layout with rooms of real-life designs. Instead they were more concerned with cognitive thinking and reasoning.

Cue Cards

The therapist would show me cue cards of different pictures of shapes, sizes, and colors. I would have to match the pictures, put them in order, or redraw the pictures like the one shown to me. Here is an example some of a cue cards.

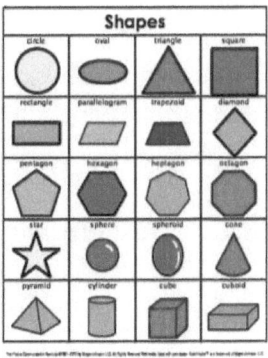

Driving Test

One day the occupational therapist inquired about my driving license. She asked if I wanted to retake the written and driving test. I replied yes! The therapist then administered the written test to me. I did sufficiently. I am not going to tell you my score. I went on to take the driving part of the test.

I didn't drive a real car, but it was like one. It was like a car game that you would buy for your video game system. But it wasn't a game. It had two doors, key ignition, seat belts, speedometer, gear shift, rearview mirror, and turn signal. The therapist

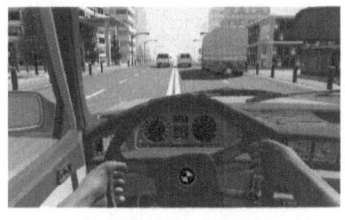

would instruct me to put on my seat belt, start the car, and put it in drive. A video was guiding me through the process.

The therapist would observe and monitor my score of traffic violations. She would detect how I responded to red lights, stop signs, trains, approaching traffic, highways, pedestrians, and distractions. My score would determine how long I was going to keep starting over and taking the driving test. I did minimal requirements. I am not going to tell you how many times I started over (LOL).

Speech Therapy

Not only did Health South and Centre for Neuro Skills Rehabilitations provide me with physical and occupational therapy, they also wanted me as a stroke patient to improve on my speech skills as well. All the therapists work together to promote me to independence.

Once a stroke survivor has taken his or her last step to go home, then it's independence (on your own with your family and friends)—trusting God and yourself; staying in the Word of God; building your spiritual, physical, and mental strength; and detoxing your mind, body, and soul.

Speech therapy consists of comprehending your reading and writing skills. Memory skills are very important, such as your social interaction like reasoning, decisions you make, and your attention span. The therapist uses retraining techniques to restore the stroke patient's skills and abilities.

There was an hour each for speech, reading, math, physical, and occupational therapy at Centre for Neuro Skills. I was there from 9:00 a.m. to 2:00 p.m. and had thirty minutes for lunch, like school. The therapist would evaluate what I read and if I circled the correct answer on the test. The therapist would maintain my progress in language and cognitive therapy. Cognitive skills testing measured my mental capacity.

Memory

Memory is retrieved information in the brain. It's what a person thinks when he or she reads or sees something. If the memory is interrupted from a stroke, this process may be temporary or permanently damaged. Some stroke patients can remember previous experiences but can't recall what happened to them this month. Memory loss is connected to cognitive and emotional process.

If a stroke patient loses concentration or attention span is slow, this will lead to depression, which hinders motivation. These will have a negative influence on your memory, for example, not having the mental ability to remember an important vacation. This is confusing to a stroke patient and will create a change in the patient. This is the reason for retraining a person.

It's concentrating on a more practical solution than just memory improvement. That's when the speech therapist comes in to interact with the stroke patient.

Impairment Skills in Speech

You must communicate for your memory to be nurtured or shaped, such as language, reading, writing, and visual. These skills are necessary in achieving independence in the real world. This is where speech therapy comes in. Language relates to speech. When it is impaired, some patients' verbal expressions become difficult. This happens in a left-brain stroke survivor.

There is a list of problems with this patient. One example is the right side is weak or paralyzed. Their hearing is not the same. Because of what they hear, they misunderstand. Speech therapy techniques are mandatory. For example, when you speak, use short sentences. Conversations should be slow and simple to a stroke patient.

At Centre for Neuro Skills, speech therapy consists of reading, language, hearing, writing, and visual. The therapist would have me read short stories and then circle the correct answer to the question at the end of the story. Other times she would have me work on math problems. I was using all my skills in speech. Some stroke patients don't understand what they have just read. They probably comprehend what they see and say the words correctly but not what they read.

The speech therapist would display various cue cards of household items, for instance, a toothbrush, lamp, sofa, table, and bed. She would tell me, "Repeat what I just displayed before you." This is where I used my memory skills. The speech therapist was testing my brain and memory skills. She would display a letter of the alphabet. I had to think of twenty-five words that begin with that letter.

For example, the letter M equals man, motor, mission, moon, music, miracle, makeup, Matthew, milk, mustache, move, muscle, and Mike, and the list goes up to twenty-five words. A stroke patient with speech problems often has problems with writing as well. The patient cannot write complete sentences or use correct grammar. The good news is that reading and writing skills can be relearned with certain techniques from the therapist.

Final Team Builders/Team Members

I have discussed the different team members in rehabilitation at Centre for Neuro Skills. A vocational specialist would evaluate my skills. She would determine if I were able to return to the job market or not, probably in a different line of work than I worked in before. The goal was to help me as a stroke patient to reenter the community with a different approach.

At Centre for Neuro Skills, a rehabilitation counselor was someone that stroke patients could go to and discuss their behavioral problems with if the patient were angry, depressed, or anxious. The case manager was concerned with one's overall well-being. If you had insurance issues or questions, she would provide names and addresses of support groups. She would work with your financial situation. These team members significantly helped me and other stroke patients with self-care and to rebuild our lives and return home and then back into the real world.

Successfully Completing Rehabilitations

Rehabilitation may not be able to bring back to life dead parched brain cells. Although rehabilitation can give you back much of what has been lost, it can give you alternative ways to live life again and move forward. At each rehabilitation, each team member is consistent with his or her routines and treatments. Each person sets realistic goals for the stroke patient. The therapist consistently reinforces lessons until the stroke patient learns them well. The therapist suggests strategies such as walkers, canes, and braces when strength and balance is affected.

Rehabilitation can encourage a stroke patient to walk, communicate, and become independent again. Not only can a stroke survivor take a function and translate it into action, if the stroke patient repeatedly does this task daily, it would redirect brain cells. Stroke patients must be encouraged to use their affected arm or leg. Doing this daily will help the patient reenter the community.

The stroke survivor will be able to function day to day by taking a shower, getting dressed, and going to the supermarket. This promotes self-esteem, confidence, and motivation. The stroke patient starts making progress every day. Depression leaves, and the stroke patient has a renewed life once again. I would like to thank my Lord and Savior, Jesus Christ; my primary physician; my neurologist; Health South; and Centre for Neuro Skills. Thank all of you for everything you have done for me.

I pray that God blesses all of you with divine health. Joel 2:25 (NIV) says, "I will repay you for the years the locusts have eaten the great locust and the young locust, the other locust and the locust swarm my great army that I sent among you."

CHAPTER 10

THINGS TO REMEMBER

Some stroke patients have physical and psychological problems after a stroke. The pain is worse after a stroke. Their sex drive has lessened. The desire is gone. They don't feel sexy. Patience runs thin in most marriages concerning stroke victims. The children feel frustrated because they must take care of their parent. They must help and support you. The children may have feelings of anger and fear.

I can discuss the physical conditions of a stroke. I can go into detail of left-brain strokes. I can pinpoint the parts of the brain that was affected. I can have outlined specific therapy programs at rehabilitations. The truth of the matter is that emotions and feelings change from day to day.

Emotions

Emotions are important in a stroke survivor's life. Emotions can affect the outcome of a stroke survivor rehabilitation program. It can become a successful or unsuccessful completion. In a stroke patient, social skills are difficult to improve, whereas physical skills are less complicated to achieve in improvement. The recreational activities will improve as time increases. Most patients don't want to accept living life after a stroke.

Major emotional issues that happen at the beginning of a stroke is shock and anger. The shock of a stroke brings about a change in a person's life. Families often sense this as being unreal. Families feel like this can't be happening. Stroke survivors finally realize that things must change in their life. For example, their life has been altered.

They try to deny it, but nevertheless, it has occurred. After the shock, then comes anger. The stroke patient asks, "Why me? This is not fair! Why? Why? Why?" The patient feels shock and anger together. The person wants an answer. So he or she starts requesting information. For instance, the individual then starts Googling answers. The patient goes to the web and types in "strokes."

Next is going through the process of rehabilitation. This is when the stroke patient starts seeking God's Word and asking him for a miracle. The only person who could really deliver a miracle is God. So it's you and God one on one, having daily conversations, hoping and praying for a miracle. A stroke patient implies, "God, if only you will allow me to walk again."

That person makes promises to God by saying, "I promise I will take care of my health and myself." The patient says, "Allow me to walk again. I will go to church every time the church door opens. I will tell everyone about you, about how you are a healer and a miracle worker." The stroke patient confesses, "I will do all of this and more all the days of my life. In Jesus's name. Amen."

The patient hopes things will go back to normal. He or she hopes things will go back to the way he or she was before the stroke.

Depression

Once reality sets in, you will come to realize that your life may never be the same. Your life is different. The old you, the you before the stroke happened, is gone. This creates depression. Taking antidepressants or seeking counseling will help. You will feel different symptoms: fatigue, crying, complaining, anxiety, guilt, and anger. In order for a stroke patient to heal, he or she would have to accept these different symptoms of depression. The patient would have to accept his or her feelings. For example, the crying, complaining, anxiety, and anger would have to be accepted.

Depression can lead to sadness or negative feelings that may cause a lack of interest in activities. The person can have the feeling of hopelessness and unimportance in a period when he or she has very little economic activity. The person can have a mental illness or a serious mental disorder. The patient could have an illness that interferes with his or her daily living or his or her lack or decrease of energy. It can also affect one's decision making.

A change in your life has happened. Maybe the stroke has slowed down your movement. You don't move as quickly as you did before. The illness can cause changes in your brain chemistry or hormone levels. The brain has a chemical imbalance. It can be treated with medication or counseling.

Hope

Hope is knowing that things will be different but could still work out, especially when your motivation starts to improve and you have completed rehabilitation. Hope brings the patient confidence and independence. The realistic hope is that you are going to get better and you are going to survive and start a renewed life. Every stroke patient goes through the process, but hope comes in during rehabilitation.

Hope anticipate knowledge; knowledge is power. A stroke patient having knowledge can conquer depression. So grab your cell phone in front of you and Google, Google, and Google away. Learn everything you can about strokes, depression, and recovery. Learn everything from this illness. Depression and sickness will have to leave and go somewhere else, but it can't stay at your house. You don't need any roommates, unless they are paying rent and not taking your money.

Social Skills

A stroke patient needs goals. Goals can motivate you and give you positive attitudes. When stroke survivors accomplish their goals, they feel so much better about themselves. A busy schedule that fills a calendar establishes a busy routine. This can give a depressed stroke patient purpose. Stroke patients who are depressed can benefit from social activities. Daily activities in their life are beneficial.

Surround yourself with people. Go to the restaurant or supermarket, or join a group. This will get you out of your comfort zone. Enjoy the sunshine, see the green grass and colorful flowers, and feel the wind blowing. This will help you enjoy life again. Encourage a stroke survivor to accept life again. Encourage a stroke survivor to accept a hobby for himself or herself.

For instance, encourage sewing, golfing, or painting. Persuade a patient to go on a vacation or a trip. A change in scenery is very important. Go to lunch with a family member or a friend. Support groups are good for a stroke patient. Enjoy entertainment once again. It is in the eye of the beholder, and laughter comes within unexpected places.

Read the Bible, a magazine, or a book. Try listening to the radio or watching television. Enroll the stroke patient in a health program, gym, fitness center, or community YMCA. Encourage the patient to play chess, checkers, bridge, Yahtzee, or scrabble, something that will improve his or her memory or problem-solving skills.

Family

Every family member sees the stroke survivor differently. Families all have the same emotions. The stroke victim needs to be respected or treated as an adult. If not, he or she will not progress successfully. The patient is still your mom or your dad, regardless of his or her stroke. Family members need to work together to create a healthy relationship and a healthy home. Everyone in the family needs to stay healthy to take care of the survivor.

Especially keep your mind healthy in order to make your life more successful, for the stroke victim and for yourself. There is a role change for sure, whereas the children or the spouse have full responsibility of taking care of the stroke survivor. A stroke is a nightmare. There are psychological changes that take place in your mind, like "What if I get sick again?" and "Will I totally depend on my family?"

A stroke will change many of your old habits and give you new ones. So that's why you must encourage yourself again and again. Stay in the Word of God daily. Encourage the stroke patient to start cooking and cleaning in the house and doing laundry again. Patience with the stroke survivor is necessary; therefore, control your temper. Try praising the person as much as possible.

Focus on the person's abilities and not his or her disabilities. Implement a positive attitude, not a negative one. Optimism is the attitude your family should present to the survivor. The key words are, "You can do it!"

Divorce

Some challenging functions come with a stroke. These three functions—impairment, disabled, and handicapped—could lead to divorce. Impairment weakens or paralyzes your arm or leg, either on the right or left side. It depends on if you had a left- or right-brain stroke. Disabled limits your movement of the paralyzed leg or arm. Therefore, you can't perform in a normal way.

Handicapped is when you have a disadvantage. It makes life more difficult. Maybe you can't work for the same business as before. Probably part of your brain or a portion of your body has been damaged. So your handicapped was formed and shaped from an impairment in your body or brain, which creates a disability.

This sometimes leads to divorce. The divorce rate in America is high. It is common in society. There is no frowning upon it in today's world. When your partner is considering divorce, first, he or she may try to look at the situation in a positive manner. Your partner may receive advice from friends, family, counselors, and pastors. All of this can't rebuild or save your marriage. You would have to take it to God in prayer.

Really it was going to end anyway. Your marriage was probably already hurting. The stroke wasn't the determining factor that provoked your partner to pursue it. The fact of the matter is that it was going to happen, regardless of a stroke or not. A stoke can only provide your partner with the ability to choose to exit out of marriage.

If you are going to file for divorce, first, consult a professional in order to prepare you and your stroke survivor emotionally.

Safety

Once the stroke survivor returns home from rehabilitation, the family should make sure that the home is safe for him or her. Keep all electrical cords tucked away. Remove all throw rugs. Provide all the rooms in the house with night lights. Consult a professional when you purchase equipment concerning the patient. You may have to modify the bathroom. All the kitchen items need to be easy to reach. Downstairs would be easier for sleeping purposes.

Rearrange the furniture. This allows the stroke survivor to move freely. Keep the environment calm and relaxed. This is your partner or your parent, not just a stroke survivor. This is a loved one, a family member. Remember that at the end of the day.

Optimistic Behavior

A stroke survivor must remain optimistic. The patient, of course, will have unpredictable behavior like hostility, aggressiveness, or anger. These behaviors could prevent progress or success, something the patient is trying to accomplish. Going back into the real world and attending a social event could possibly be hindered. The stroke patient must keep an optimistic outlook on life.

A stroke is a reality check. The stroke survivor needs to grab a hold of this and use some determination skills to persevere and accomplish his or her goals. Rehabilitation teaches a stroke patient self-awareness. Stop repeating words like *should have, could have*, or *would have*. Instead use words like *I can, I will*, and *I believe*. Myself,

I use the serenity prayer, "God, grant me the serenity to accept the things I cannot change, the courage to change the things I can, and the wisdom to know the difference. Amen!"

Things you can change include your attitude, personality, and behavior. Then change them. Things you cannot change are a stroke and an illness. Don't worry about it. Stop stressing. Trust God, and he will make everything better. Receive knowledge and wisdom about your illness. Improve yourself as much as possible and go on with life. Trust yourself in God and his Word. Seek his Word daily. Improve your mind and physical ability. Improvement equals success. In other words, you win! Praise God!

Stroke survivors need to see the glass as half full or half empty. There are two types of people: negative and positive. You guessed it. Negative people see the glass as half empty; positive people see the glass as half full. They are so negative about everything in life. Tell me how God can answer their prayers. If they don't see anything, they don't expect anything. So therefore, they stop praying.

They don't believe that life can become better with God. These people don't add to life. They take away from life. That's why their life doesn't grow and succeed. If they start having a positive attitude, then life will become better. God's Word brings positive thoughts to your mind. That's why you must remain in his Word and his Word remains in you.

Stroke patients would recover successfully if they would just stay positive while going through the process. When you stay optimistic about your illness, you win!

Life After a Stroke

There is one thing I learned from a stroke: my life has changed. It hasn't stopped. It just changed. Sometimes an illness can prevent a person from accomplishing his or her goals in life. You can persevere to pursue your goals but probably at a slower pace. That's possible. It just takes longer to finish because your brain doesn't function like before and your body movement isn't the same as before.

Your brain and body are in slow-motion movement. If you have breath, there is life, which creates hope. Don't give up. Continue to make progress with your disability. I hope this book has enlightened your brain on strokes. Remember, take care of yourself. Go see a physician once a year for a physical. Don't forget eating healthy and exercising. Take some time out of your busy schedule and pencil in God for an hour or two every day in your life. Read the Word of God daily.

These are the four major agendas you need to keep track of. This will prevent illness in your life. A healthy life is a happy life, and a happy life with God is a successful life. Remember, with God and a healthy life, you win!